DANIELLE HEARNE

Essential Oils for Beginners

Everything You Need to Begin Enhancing Your Life With Essential Oils, and the Right Recipes to Start off Your Journey to Wellness

Disclaimer: The information provided in this book is intended for general informational purposes only and should not be considered as medical advice. It is not intended to diagnose, treat, cure, or prevent any health condition, and it is not a substitute for professional medical advice, diagnosis, or treatment. Always seek the advice of your physician or other qualified health provider with any questions you may have regarding a medical condition. Never disregard professional medical advice or delay in seeking it because of information contained in this book. If you have a known allergy or sensitivity to essential oils or any specific health concerns, consult with a healthcare professional before using essential oils or following any recommendations in this book. The author and publisher disclaim any liability arising directly or indirectly from the use of the information provided.

First edition

This book was professionally typeset on Reedsy.
Find out more at reedsy.com

"Living is about capturing the essence of things"

Danielle Hearne

Contents

One

Introduction

Essential oils are a valuable life enhancing gem that should be in every household. Many people don't realize that such a small drop of oil could have such a big impact in their lives. There are many different uses for essential oils such as for health, body aches and pains, or cleaning and household freshness. This is why one of the most amazing things about essential oils is how you can open up and smell different bottles of oils and each one will make you feel a different way or put you in a different mood. Some may relax you, some may energize you and some may instantly take your stress level down a notch. When it comes to these miracle oils the possibilities are endless.

Maybe you bought this book because this is your first time using essential oils or maybe they were gifted from a friend and you know nothing about them. Have you had them sitting in a drawer unopened for a while and you're not sure what to do with them? Or maybe you use them regularly but you are not aware of what other uses they contain besides taking a quick whiff and feeling happy thoughts. My job today is to help you get the most out of every drop so that you can unlock all the wonders that these little bottles of oils have to offer.

Using Essential oils regularly can gradually transform your everyday mood and enhance your lifestyle. It may seem like a small insignificant addition to your life, and it may be hard to believe that just by smelling some oil you could possibly get the confidence to go out and seize the day or make all your worries fade away for a short period of time. There are more to these oils than what meets the eye and we are going to unlock the secrets from within.

Unraveling the Essence: What are Essential Oils?

Essential oils are nature's aromatic treasures, capturing the very essence of plants. They are volatile, concentrated compounds meticulously extracted from various parts of plants, such as leaves, stems, flowers, or roots. These oils are often referred to as "essential" because they contain the plant's unique aroma or essence, the very soul of the plant itself.

While essential oils share the word "oil" in their name, they are not true oils in the traditional sense. Unlike the fatty oils you might use in cooking or skincare, essential oils are not greasy. Instead, they are clear, often with a thin consistency. These oils are composed of unique aromatic compounds, which are responsible for their characteristic scents.

Essential oils have been used for thousands of years in various cultures for their remarkable properties. They serve multiple purposes, from promoting relaxation and improving mood to supporting overall well-being. Many people use essential oils in aromatherapy, massage, and even for cleaning and personal care products. These oils are known for their versatility, with each type offering its own set of potential benefits.

Two

The History of Essential Oils

Essential oils have been used for centuries across various cultures, from the Egyptians to the Greeks and Romans. Evidence suggests that the Egyptians were among the first to use aromatic oils as early as 4500 B.C for both spiritual and cosmetic purposes.

The Greeks, with their rich tradition in medicine, recognized the therapeutic properties of these oils. The famous physician Hippocrates, often called the father of medicine, was known to have used aromatic oils in his practice.

The Romans, known for their elaborate bathing rituals, used essential oils in their baths for their aromatic properties and for promoting overall well-being.

Essential oils also played a significant role in traditional Chinese and Indian medicine.In traditional Chinese medicine, aromatic oils were used to balance the harmony between the individual and the cosmic forces.

In Ayurveda, the 5000-year-old Indian medicinal system, essential oils were used to balance the three fundamental doshas (life forces): Vata, Pitta, and Kapha.

The use of essential oils spread to the Arab world during the Golden Age of Islam. Ibn Sina, or Avicenna, a prominent Persian physician, is credited with the invention of the steam distillation method, which is still widely used today for extracting essential oils.Some of the first distilled oils produced were rosemary, cinnamon, sage and cedarwood. There was not very much understanding of how these oils really worked during this time.

It was during the early 1900s that chemists really started to take an interest in the development of essential oils and worked on unlocking all the secrets that they had to offer. These advancements in knowledge led to a drastic expansion in production and ignited their newfound uses in beverages, foods and perfumes.

How Essential Oils are Made:

The process of making essential oils is truly fascinating. The most common method for extracting these precious oils is through distillation, and it's a process that requires both science and artistry. Imagine a large still, not unlike those used for making spirits, but with a focus on capturing the volatile oils of plants. In steam distillation, steam is passed through a large hopper that contains raw plant materials, and this causes the aromatic compounds to be released. The steam and plant vapors and then condensed together and create a liquid. After they are cooled, the water and oil are separated. The water portion contains parts of the plant's essence, which is now called floral water or hydrosol. The oil soluble aromatic compounds rise to the top of the water, where they are then extracted and this is how pure essential oil is created and gathered.

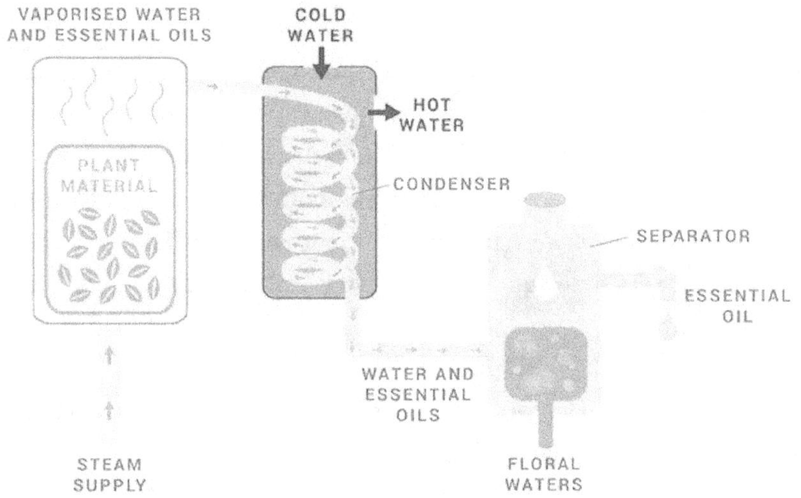

Voilà, we have our essential oil! The oils can actually be captured from a variety of plants, flowers, seeds, berries, fruits or even woods, but not all plants are suitable for this method. Some plant materials don't contain enough essential oil to make the process worthwhile. For example, imagine trying to distill essential oil from a watermelon. It's mostly water, so the yield would be negligible. Similarly, plants with very low oil content, like cotton or oak, aren't suitable candidates for essential oil extraction.

On the other hand, plants with a high oil content, like lavender or eucalyptus, are ideal choices. Their concentrated essential oils can be effectively extracted through distillation, making them valuable resources for aromatherapy, perfumery, and more. It's a difficult process to extract the oils and requires delicate treatment of its sources in order to keep its quality intact.

Understanding the right plants and the distillation process is crucial to harnessing the goodness of essential oils. It's a blend of science and nature, resulting in fragrant, concentrated elixirs.

Three

How to Use Essential Oils

The most popular and well known use would be aromatherapy which is using essential oils for therapeutic benefits. When you inhale, each scent molecule travels from the olfactory nerve directly to the brain with the main impact being on the amygdala, which is the emotional center of the brain.

Aromatherapy has been around for thousands of years and has been used for both medical and religious purposes. Only recently has it gained more traction and recognition in the fields of science and medicine. The actual term "aromatherapy" was created by a French Perfumer and chemist named Rene-Maurice Gattefosse who wrote and published a book about their medicinal benefits back in 1937. His book talks about the use of essential oils in treating medical conditions such as lavender for burn wounds.

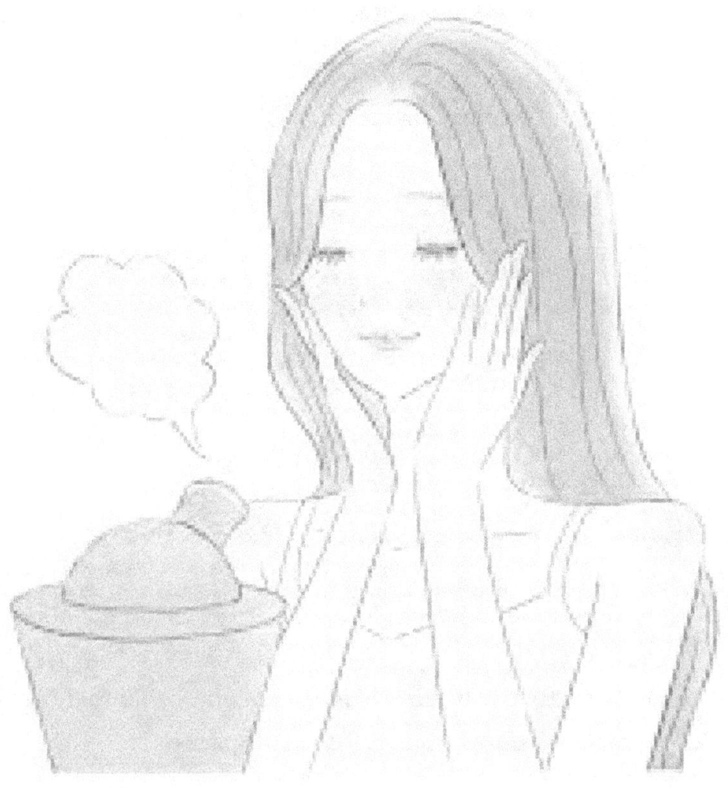

To receive benefits from aromatherapy, there are several different routes of delivery that can be used, which i will list below:

Diffusers

Essential Oil diffusers bring a sense of tranquility to any space. This is a minimal effort self-care option that can give you hours of easier breathing. The way it works is that the diffuser breaks down essential oils into smaller molecules and disperses them into the air for a pleasant and calming effect. It is the diffuser's job to make sure the particles are dispersed at a comfortable concentration that does not overbear the room. There are several different kinds of oil diffusers.

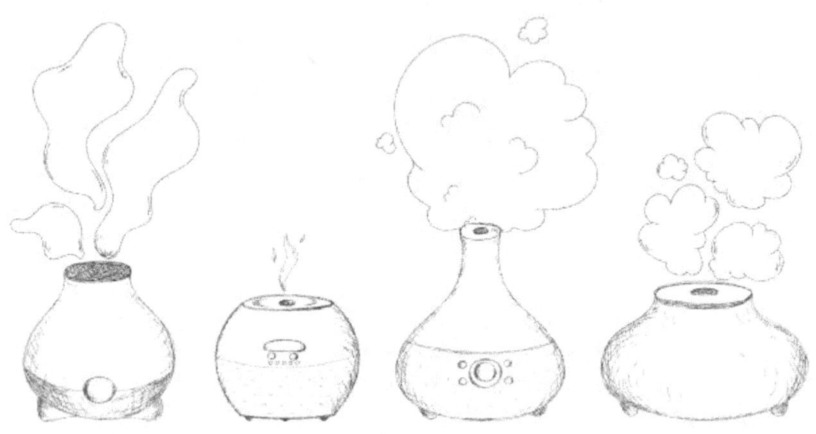

One is an evaporative diffuser. This type uses the wind to disperse the scent of essential oils. It is perfect for small spaces.

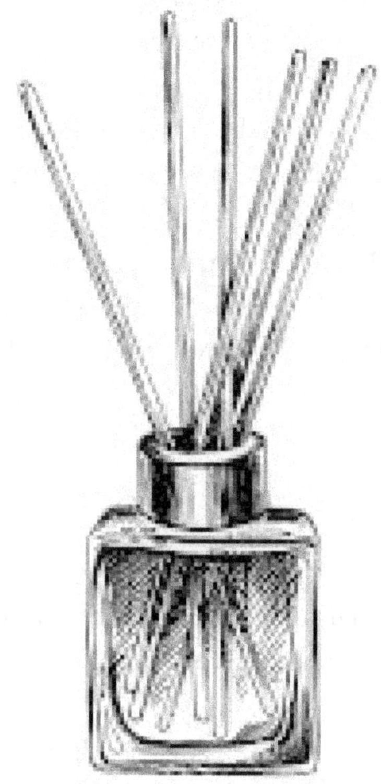

Another is inhalers. Essential oils are commonly used with various types of inhalers, each designed to cater to different preferences and needs. The primary types include:

- **Personal Inhalers:** These are small, portable devices that allow individuals to enjoy the benefits of essential oils discreetly. Personal inhalers typically consist of a compact tube with a wick or pad that holds the essential oil blend. Users can inhale directly from the device, making them perfect for on-the-go aromatherapy.

- **Nasal Inhalers:** Specifically designed for nasal application, these inhalers target the olfactory senses directly. They often feature a twist-up design, making them easy to use and convenient for precise inhalation. Nasal inhalers are commonly used for targeted aromatherapy applications, such as stress relief or mood enhancement

- **Inhalation Patches:** These innovative patches contain a blend of essential oils and are worn on the skin. The oils slowly evaporate, allowing users to benefit from inhalation throughout the day. Inhalation patches are discreet and offer a continuous aroma experience

Facial steamers: Facial steamers offer a wonderful way to enhance your skincare routine with essential oils. Here's a simple guide:

1. **Choose Your Essential Oil:** Select oils based on your skincare needs. For example, lavender for relaxation, tea tree for acne, or eucalyptus for a refreshing feel.

2. **Prepare the Steamer:** Fill your facial steamer with water. For every 100ml, add 3-5 drops of your chosen essential oil. This ratio ensures a pleasant and not overpowering aroma.

3. **Steam Settings:** Turn on the steamer and allow it to produce steam. Adjust the intensity according to your comfort.

4. **Enjoy the Steam:** Position your face at a comfortable distance, allowing the steam to open up your pores. Breathe deeply to experience the therapeutic benefits of the essential oils. start with a shorter steaming session and gradually increase the time based on your skin's response. Be sure to complete Your skincare Routine after steaming to lock in the benefits.

Aromatic Spritzers: An aromatic spritzer is a scented spray made by combining essential oils with a liquid base, often water or a water-alcohol mix. This mixture is then sprayed into the air or onto surfaces to impart a pleasant aroma to the environment. They are commonly used for various purposes, including creating a soothing ambiance, freshening up living spaces, or even as a personal fragrance. The essential oils used in spritzers can be chosen based on personal preference or desired therapeutic benefits. Popular choices include lavender for relaxation, citrus blends for a refreshing atmosphere, or peppermint for an energizing effect. Aromatic spritzers offer a convenient and versatile way to enjoy the aromatic properties of essential oils in homes, offices, or on the go.

Humidifiers: A humidifier is a device designed to increase humidity levels in the air by emitting water vapor. It is commonly used to alleviate dry skin, nasal congestion, and other respiratory issues caused by low humidity.

As for using essential oils with a humidifier, it largely depends on the type of humidifier. While some humidifiers are specifically designed to be used with essential oils, others may not be suitable. Adding essential oils to a humidifier can enhance the air with pleasant fragrances and potentially offer aromatherapeutic benefits.

However, it's crucial to follow the manufacturer's guidelines. Using essential oils in a humidifier not designed for them may damage the device or pose safety risks. If a humidifier is labeled as "essential oil-compatible" or has a designated tray or compartment for oils, it is generally safe to use them together. Always dilute essential oils properly and avoid overuse to prevent damage to the humidifier and ensure a safe and effective experience.

Oil burners: An oil burner is a device used to diffuse fragrant oils into the air, creating a pleasant aroma. It typically consists of a bowl or dish to hold the oils and a heat source beneath to vaporize them. The heat source can be a tea light candle or an electric element.

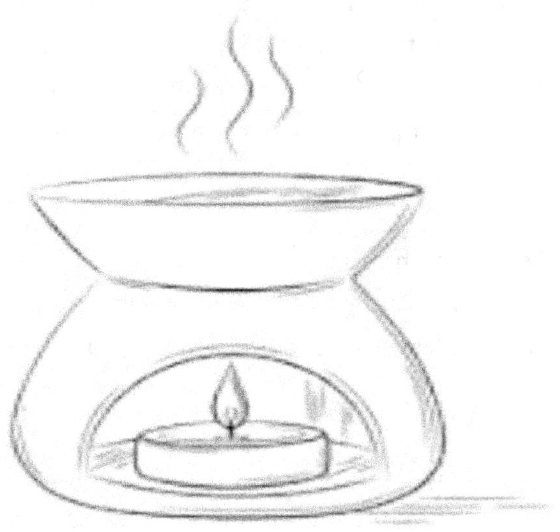

When using an oil burner, you don't burn essential oils in the traditional sense; instead, you heat them to release their aroma. Place a few drops of essential oil into the bowl or dish of the oil burner, and as the heat source warms the oil, it evaporates into the air, filling the space with the desired scent.

Four

Categories and Types of Essential Oils

Essential oils exhibit a diverse array of aromas, allowing them to be categorized based on their scent profiles, with each category presenting unique olfactory experiences and potential benefits.

The citrus category encompasses oils like lemon, orange, and grapefruit, renowned for their refreshing and uplifting scents that often promote energy and a positive mood.

In the floral category, oils such as lavender, rose, and chamomile offer sweet, delicate, and sometimes powdery aromas, making them popular choices for relaxation and emotional balance.

Oils like rosemary, basil, and thyme fall into the herbaceous category, emitting fresh, green, and slightly spicy scents that contribute to mental clarity and focus.

The woody category includes oils like cedarwood, sandalwood, and pine, characterized by warm, earthy, and grounding aromas that foster a sense of stability and calm.

Minty oils, including peppermint and spearmint, provide invigorating and cool fragrances, often used to promote revitalization and alertness.

In the spicy category, oils like cinnamon, clove, and ginger offer warm, rich, and sometimes exotic aromas associated with a cozy and comforting ambiance.

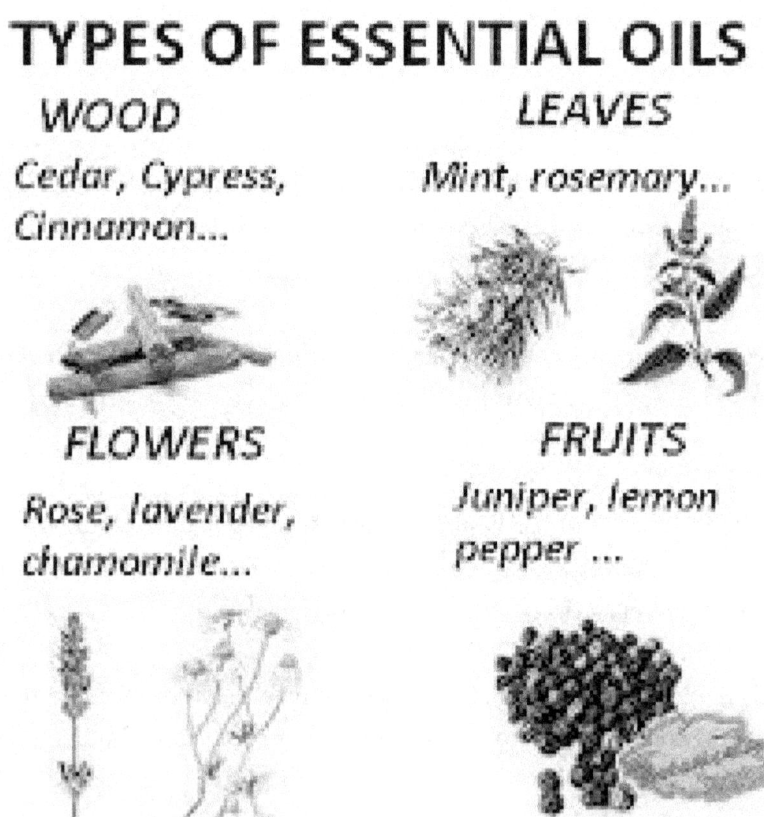

Recognizing these aroma categories empowers individuals to select essential oils that align with their preferences and the specific ambiance they aim to create, be it one of relaxation, energy, or focus.

Types of oils and their uses:

Floral oils: Floral essential oils are plant-derived oils extracted from the flowers of various plants. These oils capture the aromatic compounds of flowers, offering a range of distinct and pleasant scents.

The Calming Trio: Lavender, Chamomile, and Ylang Ylang

Lavender oil is renowned for its calming properties, making it an ideal choice for promoting relaxation and aiding in sleep. Whether diffused in your bedroom or added to a carrier oil for a soothing massage, its versatile application allows you to incorporate it into your nightly routine. For a quick stress-relief fix during the day, a few drops in a diffuser can create a serene atmosphere. Additionally, lavender oil's gentle nature makes it suitable for addressing minor skin irritations, providing a natural solution for soothing skin discomfort. According to research by the National Library of Medicine, lavender oil has shown potential in treating anxiety, depression, and restlessness.

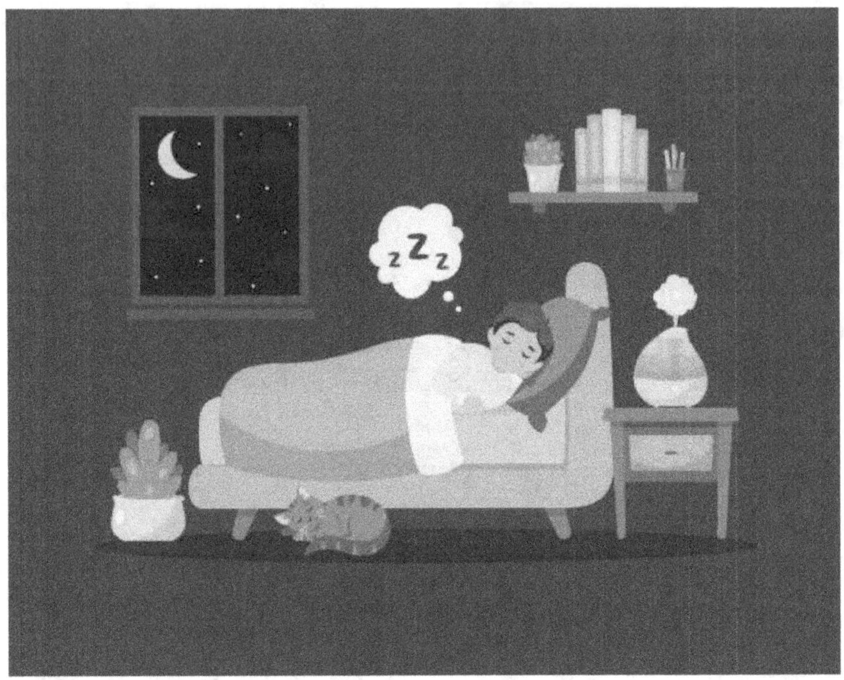

Chamomile oil boasts a myriad of health benefits that can enhance your well-being. Known for its calming properties, it can be your go-to remedy for stress relief and promoting a restful sleep. Additionally, chamomile oil is celebrated for its anti-inflammatory and soothing effects, making it a gentle yet effective solution for skin irritations and conditions. Whether inhaled through aromatherapy or applied topically, chamomile oil stands as a versatile ally in nurturing both your mental and physical health.

Ylang Ylang oil, is a powerhouse with diverse health benefits. Known for its floral and sweet fragrance, Ylang Ylang is cherished for its ability to reduce stress and anxiety, promoting a sense of calm and relaxation. This exotic oil is also recognized for its potential to balance and regulate mood, making it a natural mood enhancer. Beyond its emotional benefits, Ylang Ylang oil is thought to have aphrodisiac properties and may contribute to skin health. Whether diffused, applied topically, or incorporated into your beauty routine, Ylang Ylang oil adds a touch of exotic luxury to your holistic well-being journey.

Jasmine Oil is loved for its exotic, floral scent. It is often used in aromatherapy for its mood-lifting and aphrodisiac properties. Research suggests that jasmine oil can uplift your mood and enhance romantic feelings. Jasmine oil can be added to homemade body lotions or massage oils for a luxurious self-care routine.

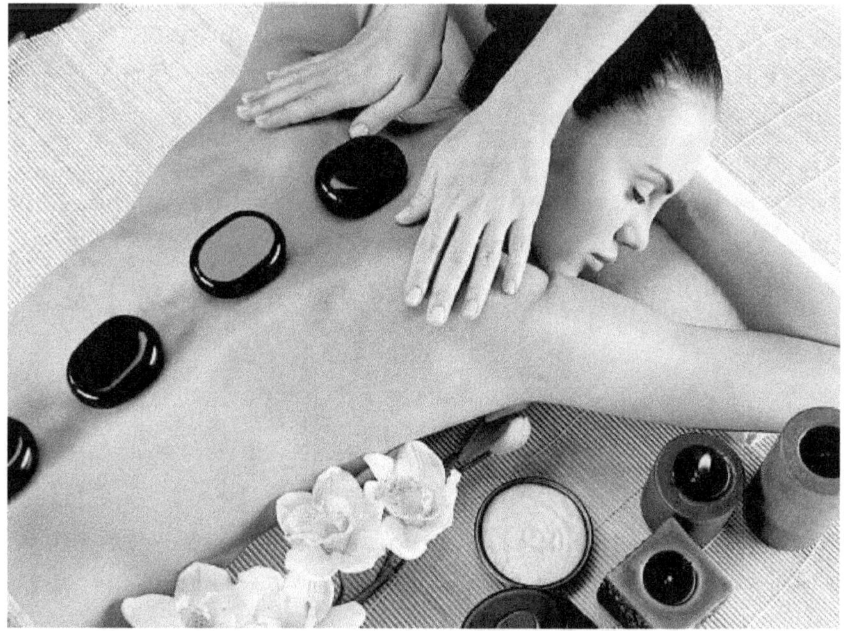

The Energizers: Peppermint, Rosemary and Lemon

Peppermint oil is a versatile essential oil known for its invigorating properties. Its refreshing scent makes it an excellent choice to boost your energy, focus and uplift your mood. Add a few drops to a diffuser for a revitalizing aroma in your workspace or mix it with a carrier oil for a refreshing massage. Peppermint oil can also be a natural solution for occasional headaches when applied topically to the temples, and can be applied topically to relieve muscle pain when diluted with a carrier oil. Its been reported that peppermint oil can enhance memory and increase alertness. Keep this dynamic oil on hand for a quick and effective pick-me-up throughout the day.

Rosemary Oil, often associated with memory and focus, is used in aromatherapy to enhance mental clarity and concentration, and has also been said to improve cognitive performance. Rosemary oil is also commonly used in hair care routines, as it's believed to stimulate hair growth and reduce dandruff

Lemon Oil has an invigorating and citrusy scent. It is often used to uplift the mood and boost energy levels. Lemon oil is also popular in homemade cleaning products due to its antibacterial properties and fresh scent.

Lets talk about citrus oils:
Incorporating a variety of citrus oils allows you to tailor your aromatherapy experience to different moods and occasions. Whether you're seeking invigoration, relaxation, or a bright atmosphere, these citrus oils offer a delightful range of options.

Alongside the familiar zest of lemon, there's the sweet and fruity embrace of orange oil, radiating warmth and positivity. Grapefruit oil offers a slightly tangy scent that promotes a sense of vitality and freshness, while lime oil adds a zesty and energizing twist to your aromatic repertoire. Derived from the bergamot orange, bergamot oil introduces a citrusy, floral aroma, celebrated for its calming properties and stress-alleviating potential. For a soothing touch, mandarin oil contributes a sweet and gentle fragrance, perfect for creating a comforting atmosphere.

Orange Oil: Radiating warmth and positivity, orange oil offers a sweet and fruity aroma. It's often used to uplift the spirits and add a cheerful note to blends.

Grapefruit Oil: With its invigorating and slightly tangy scent, grapefruit oil is a popular choice for promoting a sense of vitality and freshness. It's also recognized for its potential benefits for skin health.

Lime Oil: Bursting with a zesty and energizing fragrance, lime oil adds a vibrant twist. It's commonly used to enhance mood and create a lively atmosphere.

Mandarin Oil: Known for its sweet and gentle aroma, mandarin oil is a soothing option that can promote relaxation. It's often used in blends for its comforting qualities.

The Healers: Tea Tree, Eucalyptus, and Frankincense

Tea Tree: renowned for its potent health benefits. This essential oil is a stalwart in skincare, known for its powerful antibacterial and anti-inflammatory properties. Tea tree oil is a go-to solution for treating acne, soothing skin irritations, and promoting a clear complexion. Additionally, its antifungal qualities make it effective in addressing various skin conditions. Whether applied topically or incorporated into homemade skincare products, tea tree oil stands as a natural powerhouse for skin health and overall well-being.

Eucalyptus: Widely recognized for its respiratory support, eucalyptus oil can help alleviate congestion and promote easier breathing. Its antimicrobial properties make it a valuable ally during the cold and flu season. When diffused, eucalyptus oil not only clears the air but also contributes to a revitalizing atmosphere. Whether inhaled or applied topically with a carrier oil, this powerhouse oil offers a refreshing and health-promoting addition to your well-being toolkit.

Frankincense: This oil has many benefits.

1. ***Skin Health:*** When diluted and applied topically, frankincense oil may support skin health, helping to reduce the appearance of blemishes and promoting a radiant complexion.
2. ***Stress Relief:*** The calming and grounding aroma of frankincense oil has been associated with stress relief and relaxation, making it a popular choice for aromatherapy and meditation.
3. ***Respiratory Support:*** Inhaling the vapor of frankincense oil may provide respiratory support, helping to clear the airways and promote easier breathing.
4. ***Anti-Inflammatory Properties:*** Frankincense oil contains compounds with potential anti-inflammatory properties, which could be beneficial for addressing minor inflammation.
5. ***Emotional Well-Being:*** Some users find that the aroma of frankincense oil has mood-enhancing qualities, promoting emotional well-being and a sense of tranquility.

It's important to note that while frankincense oil has been traditionally used for various purposes, individual responses may vary, and it's advisable to patch-test and consult with a healthcare professional if you have specific concerns or conditions.

I hope you now have a clear understanding of different essential oils, their unique properties, and practical uses. This will empower you to choose the right oils for your needs and incorporate them into your everyday life confidently.

Carriers, Diffusers and Blends:

We also have diluted oils, which is when the essential oil is mixed in with a carrier oil. These are more commonly used topically on the skin because essential oils by themselves are potent and can cause irritation when applied to the skin directly. Most carrier oils have little to no scent so they don't interfere with the essential oil's therapeutic properties. Some examples of carrier oils may be coconut oil, almond oil, avocado oil, grapeseed oil, olive oil, sunflower oil or rosehip oil.

Carrier oils play a crucial role in the world of essential oils, serving as a base to dilute potent essential oils before topical application. This dilution is essential to minimize skin sensitivity and avoid potential irritation. Popular choices for carrier oils include coconut oil, known for its moisturizing properties; jojoba oil, which closely resembles the skin's natural oils; and almond oil, appreciated for its mild and hypoallergenic nature. For instance, if you're drawn to lavender oil for its calming benefits and wish to apply it to your skin, it is advisable to dilute it with a carrier oil. This not only ensures a safe application but also enhances the spreadability of the essential oil, allowing you to enjoy its aromatic and therapeutic effects without compromising skin comfort. Understanding the role of carrier oils in essential oil application is a key element in promoting a positive and safe experience.

Blends are a dynamic fusion of different essential oils, and are crafted to achieve specific effects and can be applied through a diffuser, with a carrier oil on the skin, or simply inhaled from the bottle. Consider a blend designed to invigorate and boost focus, where peppermint oil brings an energizing kick, rosemary oil contributes mental clarity, and a hint of lemon oil adds a refreshing zing. This combination, whether diffused in your workspace or applied topically, exemplifies how blends can be tailored to suit your needs, offering a personalized and effective way to integrate the benefits of essential oils into your daily routine.

When aiming for a restful night's sleep, a blend may include lavender oil for its calming properties, chamomile oil to enhance its soothing effects, and sweet orange oil to introduce a touch of uplifting aroma. The versatility of blends allows you to tailor your aromatic experience according to your needs and preferences, providing a dynamic and personalized approach to enjoying the benefits of essential oils.

Five

Safety Is No Accident: Navigating Essential Oils with Care

Understanding Dilution: The Art of Mixing Essential Oils

Using essential oils safely is key to enjoying their benefits without any adverse effects. From understanding dilution to recognizing potential allergens, this chapter will walk you through everything you need to know to use essential oils safely.

Dilution emerges as a crucial step in the safe and effective utilization of essential oils. This process involves blending essential oils with carrier oils, ensuring a reduction in potency while preserving their inherent benefits. For instance, when considering a skin treatment with tea tree oil, the direct application is not recommended. Instead, you dilute a few drops of tea tree oil with a tablespoon of a carrier oil such as sweet almond oil. This careful mixture not only mitigates the risk of skin sensitivity but also facilitates even application, allowing you to harness the therapeutic properties of tea tree oil without compromising your skin's well-being. Understanding and practicing proper dilution is a fundamental aspect of incorporating essential oils into your daily self-care routine.

The correct dilution ratio is a crucial consideration, and it can vary based on the specific essential oil and its intended purpose. Generally, a recommended dilution rate falls within the range of 1% to 2% for most applications. This translates to adding approximately 6 to 12 drops of essential oil to one ounce of carrier oil. For instance, if you're preparing a skin treatment using tea tree oil, adhering to this dilution guideline is vital. By mixing a few drops of tea tree oil with a tablespoon of sweet almond oil, you not only achieve the desired dilution but also promote safe and effective application, minimizing the risk of skin sensitivity. Adopting the appropriate dilution ratio ensures that you can seamlessly integrate the benefits of essential oils into your daily self-care routine with confidence and precision.

It's crucially important to recognize that the correct dilution ratio is not only about safety but also about optimizing the benefits of essential oils. While there might be variations in the recommended dilution depending on the essential oil and its intended purpose, it's essential to note that a higher dilution doesn't equate to greater benefits. In fact, using essential oils undiluted can pose risks, such as skin irritation and other unwanted reactions. The delicate balance lies in achieving a dilution that enhances the efficacy of the essential oil while ensuring the well-being of your skin.

For most applications, a dilution rate of 1% to 2% is the widely suggested range, striking the right balance between potency and safety. This means incorporating about 6 to 12 drops of essential oil into one ounce of carrier oil. When creating a blend or preparing for a specific application, adhering to this guideline ensures that you can enjoy the full therapeutic potential of essential oils without compromising skin comfort. By understanding the importance of proper dilution, you not only safeguard against potential adverse effects but also optimize the positive impact of essential oils in your daily wellness routine. Remember, it's the thoughtful combination of potency and safety that allows you to harness the true essence of these powerful natural extracts.

Recognizing Potential Allergens: Not Every Oil is for Everyone

Just like with any other product, some people might be allergic to certain essential oils. Knowing how to recognize potential allergens can help prevent adverse reactions. For instance, if you're allergic to citrus fruits, you might want to avoid citrus oils like lemon or grapefruit.

Conducting a patch test before using a new essential oil can help identify any potential allergic reactions. To do a patch test, apply a small amount of the diluted essential oil to a patch of skin and wait for 24 hours to see if any reaction occurs. Conducting a patch test before incorporating a new essential oil into your routine adds an additional layer of precaution, helping to pinpoint any potential allergic reactions or sensitivities. This straightforward test involves applying a small amount of the diluted essential oil to a patch of skin, preferably on the inner forearm or wrist, and then waiting for a 24-hour period to observe any reactions. This precautionary step is especially significant as individual responses to essential oils can vary, and what suits one person may not be suitable for another. By dedicating a small area for the patch test, you can swiftly identify any adverse reactions before widespread application.

This prudent approach ensures that you can enjoy the benefits of essential oils without the risk of unexpected skin sensitivities, allowing for a more personalized and tailored integration into your self-care routine.If you have a known allergy or are prone to allergic reactions, it's a good idea to consult with a healthcare provider before using essential oils.

Essential Oils and Children: What Parents Need to Know

While essential oils can be beneficial for people of all ages, they should be used cautiously with children. Here's what you need to remember.

- Some essential oils, like eucalyptus and peppermint, can be over-powering for children and should be avoided. Instead, opt for kid-friendly oils like lavender and chamomile.
- Always use a higher dilution ratio when using essential oils with children. A safe dilution ratio is generally 0.5% to 1%, which is about 3 to 6 drops of essential oil per ounce of carrier oil.
- Never leave essential oils within reach of children. They can be harmful or fatal if swallowed.

Essential Oils and Pets: A Word of Caution

- Pets, especially cats and dogs, can be sensitive to essential oils. Here's what you need to consider before using essential oils around your pets.
- Some essential oils, such as tea tree, citrus, and ylang-ylang, can be toxic to pets and should be avoided.
- Always diffuse essential oils in a well-ventilated area and make sure your pet has the option to leave the room if they want to.
- Before applying any essential oils to your pet, consult with a vet. What is safe for humans might not be safe for pets.

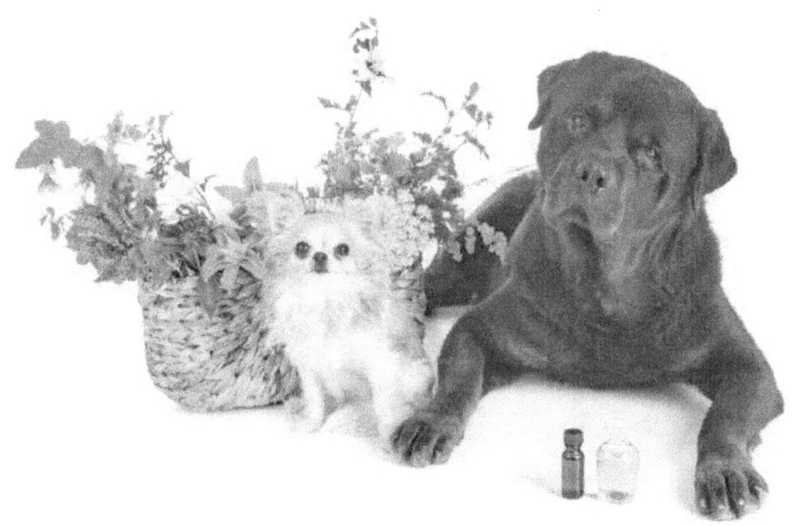

When Things Go Wrong: Handling Adverse Reactions

Even when used correctly, essential oils can sometimes cause adverse reactions. Knowing how to handle these situations can help prevent panic and further complications.

If an essential oil causes skin irritation, apply a carrier oil to the area to dilute the essential oil and alleviate the irritation. Avoid using water as it can drive the oil further into the skin.If an essential oil is ingested accidentally, contact poison control immediately. Don't induce vomiting unless instructed to do so by a healthcare professional. If you experience any unusual symptoms after using essential oils, like dizziness, nausea, or a rash, stop using the oil and seek medical advice.

By using essential oils safely and responsibly, you can enjoy their numerous benefits without any worries. Always remember, when it comes to essential oils, less is often more.

The Uncharted Territory: Exploring Lesser-Known Essential Oils

Prepare to broaden your aromatic horizons, encouraging exploration and experimentation as we uncover the properties and potential benefits of these less mainstream, but equally impactful essential oils. This exploration not only expands your knowledge but also invites you to experiment, enhancing your well-being journey with these distinct and beneficial aromatic gems.

Neroli Oil: The Understated Powerhouse

Neroli oil, derived from the blossoms of the bitter orange tree, is packed with potential benefits that are often overlooked.Neroli oil has been found to have a calming effect on the body and mind, making it a great aid for those dealing with stress and anxiety. It can also promote a positive mood and is often used in aromatherapy sessions aiming to boost happiness and well-being. Additionally, Neroli oil possesses strong antimicrobial properties, making it useful in natural cleaning products and personal care items

Vetiver Oil: The Hidden Gem

Vetiver oil, distilled from the roots of the vetiver plant, is a rich, earthy oil that's been under the radar for too long. Known for its grounding properties, vetiver oil can help promote a sense of calm and stability, and is often used in meditation practices. It has also been studied for its potential effects on attention and focus, with promising results. Vetiver oil is incredibly moisturizing and can be a great addition to DIY skincare routines, especially for those with dry or mature skin.

Copaiba Oil: The Unsung Hero

Copaiba oil, sourced from the resin of the copaiba tree, is another lesser-known essential oil with a host of potential benefits. It is known for its anti-inflammatory properties and has been used in traditional medicine for pain relief. Copaiba oil also has potential benefits for skin health and can help soothe irritated or acne-prone skin. Additionally, it has a warm, woodsy aroma that can make a lovely addition to homemade candle or soap recipes.

Clary Sage Oil: The Overlooked All-Rounder

Clary sage oil, extracted from the clary sage plant, is a versatile oil that deserves more recognition. It is often used for its calming effects and can help alleviate feelings of stress and anxiety. Clary sage oil can also help promote a good night's sleep and is a popular choice for bedtime diffuser blends. Plus, it has been studied for its potential benefits for women's health, particularly in relieving menstrual discomfort

By exploring these lesser-known essential oils, you can expand your toolkit and discover new ways to improve your health and well-being. Always remember to use them safely, and don't be afraid to experiment and find what works best for you. The world of essential oils is vast and full of potential, and it's yours to explore.

Seven

Buying Smart and Storing Right: Your Guide to Quality Essential Oils

This Chapter is your guide to savvy essential oil shopping and effective storage practices. To empower yourself with the knowledge to make informed purchasing decisions, you must learn the markers of high-quality, pure essential oils. You must also know how to store your essential oils correctly, ensuring their potency remains intact for maximum effectiveness. Get ready to become a discerning essential oil enthusiast, equipped with the skills to preserve the purity and power of your oils.

Sniffing Out the Genuine: How to Identify Pure Essential Oils

When shopping for essential oils, there are many different varieties as well as quality. Quality can range from pure and concentrated to synthetic oils, which contain little to no natural ingredients in them.

Authentic essential oils are highly concentrated and shouldn't feel oily or greasy to the touch, unlike vegetable oils. For instance, if you place a drop of a pure essential oil like eucalyptus or tea tree on a piece of paper, it will evaporate completely without leaving an oily residue. Conversely, synthetic oils or oils diluted with vegetable oils will leave a greasy stain on the paper.

Reliable brands provide complete information about their oils. Look for Latin names, country of origin, method of extraction, and part of the plant used.For example, a high-quality lavender oil might be labeled as "Lavandula angustifolia, steam distilled from flowers, grown in France."If this information is missing or vague, it might be a sign that the oil isn't pure or high quality.

Price can also be an indicator of quality. High-quality essential oils are costly to produce, so if an oil is significantly cheaper than others, it might not be pure. For example, rose oil is one of the most expensive essential oils due to the number of rose petals required for each drop of oil. If you find a full-sized bottle of rose oil for a low price, it's probably not pure.

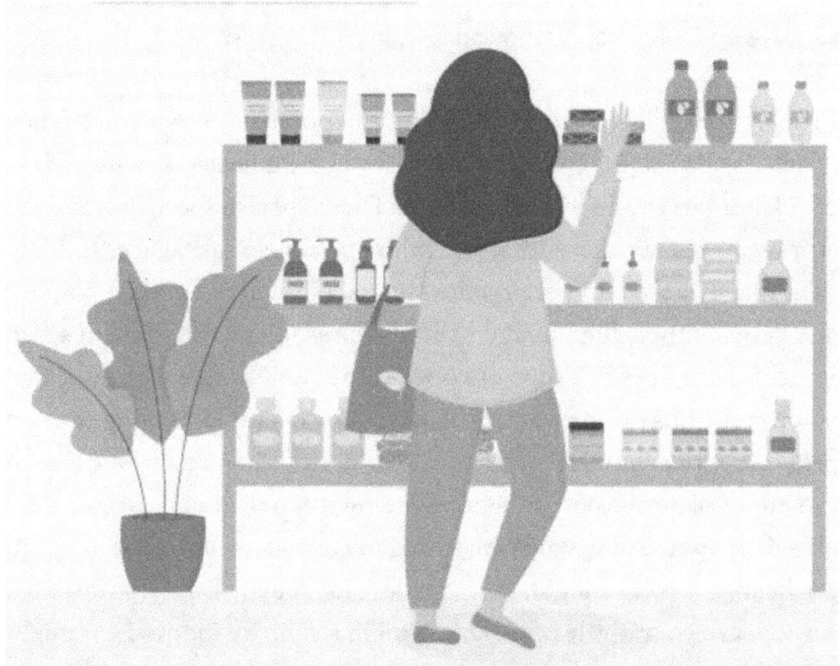

The Right Package: Understanding the Importance of Bottling and Labeling.

Essential oils should always be sold in dark-colored glass bottles to protect them from light, which can speed up oxidation and degrade the oil. Amber and cobalt blue are the most common colors, but green and violet are also acceptable.

Shelf Life and Storage: Ensuring Your Essential Oils Last Longer

Essential oils have a shelf life and can go bad. Knowing the typical lifespan of your oils can help you use them at their best and avoid using them once they've gone bad. Citrus oils like lemon and grapefruit have the shortest shelf life, typically 1-2 years. Floral and herbaccous oils like lavender and rosemary can last 4-5 years, while woodsy oils like sandalwood and cedarwood can last up to 10 years.

Proper storage is key to maintaining the potency of your oils. They should be stored in a cool, dark place, away from heat and light. A dark cabinet or box is a good storage place. There are also specially designed storage boxes out there for those who don't have safe spaces to store their oils. If stored properly, your essential oils will retain their potency and provide their therapeutic benefits for as long as possible. It's also important to keep the caps of your essential oil bottles tightly sealed when not in use to prevent oxidation. For example, leaving the cap off your peppermint oil bottle for long periods can result in a loss of the menthol aroma component, reducing its cooling and invigorating effects. If your essential oils are stored in clear glass or plastic, or left in the heat or direct sunlight, they can degrade much faster. For instance, if you leave your bottle of rosemary oil in a sunny windowsill, it might lose its potency within a few months.

With this guide, even beginners can confidently buy high-quality essential oils and keep them in optimal condition for as long as possible, ensuring they get the most out of each drop.

Eight

Everyday Magic: Integrating Essential Oils into Your Daily Routine

In the upcoming section, our focus shifts to practical integration, providing beginners with a roadmap to seamlessly weave essential oils into their daily routines. From elevating personal care rituals and household cleaning to offering stress relief and promoting overall well-being, essential oils emerge as versatile companions, poised to enhance the quality of everyday life. Let's explore how these aromatic wonders can become an integral part of your daily activities, promoting a harmonious and fragrant lifestyle.

Personal Care with Essential Oils:

Essential oils can greatly enhance your personal care routine. Tea Tree Oil, known for its antibacterial properties making it an effective addition to homemade face masks or cleansers.

Bergamot Oil has been used to reduce inflammation and promote skin regeneration, making it a beneficial addition to homemade body lotions.

Essential oils can also be incorporated into hair care. Rosemary oil, for example, is known to promote hair growth and can be added to homemade hair masks or oils.A simple hair care recipe could include mixing a few drops of Rosemary Oil with a carrier oil like jojoba oil, and applying it to the scalp.

Oral care can also benefit from the use of essential oils. Peppermint oil is a common addition to homemade toothpaste for its refreshing flavor and antibacterial properties. A homemade toothpaste recipe could include baking soda, coconut oil, and a few drops of peppermint oil.

Essential Oils for a Clean Home

Essential oils can be used to make natural and effective household cleaners. For example, Lemon and Pine oils are known for their powerful cleaning properties. Lemon oil, combined with vinegar makes a potent and eco-friendly kitchen cleaner. Pine oil can be used to create a refreshing and antiseptic floor cleaner.

Essential oils can also be used to freshen up laundry. Adding a few drops of Lavender or Chamomile oil to wool dryer balls can leave your clothes smelling fresh without any artificial fragrances.

Lavender oil is known for its calming scent which can give your clothes a soothing aroma.

Chamomile oil imparts a light, comforting scent to your laundry.

Soothing the Mind: Essential Oils for Stress Relief

Essential oils can be a powerful tool for stress relief. Since Lavender and Ylang Ylang are known for their calming properties, they can be diffused in the home or applied topically for a relaxing effect, and can even help you fall asleep in the evening.

A simple stress relief blend can be made by combining Ylang Ylang with a carrier oil like coconut oil and applying it to the wrists or temples.

Essential oils can also be incorporated into a relaxing bath routine. Adding a few drops of Eucalyptus or Frankincense oil to bath water can create a spa-like experience at home.Eucalyptus oil, is known for its invigorating scent that can help clear the mind after a long day.

Frankincense oil has a grounding aroma that can help reduce feelings of anxiety and promote relaxation.

Everyday Wellness: Essential Oils for Health:

Essential oils can be used to support everyday health and well-being. For instance, Ginger and Peppermint oils are known to help with digestion and can be used in a massage oil or taken internally with proper guidance. A digestive support blend can be made by combining Ginger oil with a carrier oil and massaging it onto the stomach while peppermint oil can be added to a glass of water after meals to support digestion.

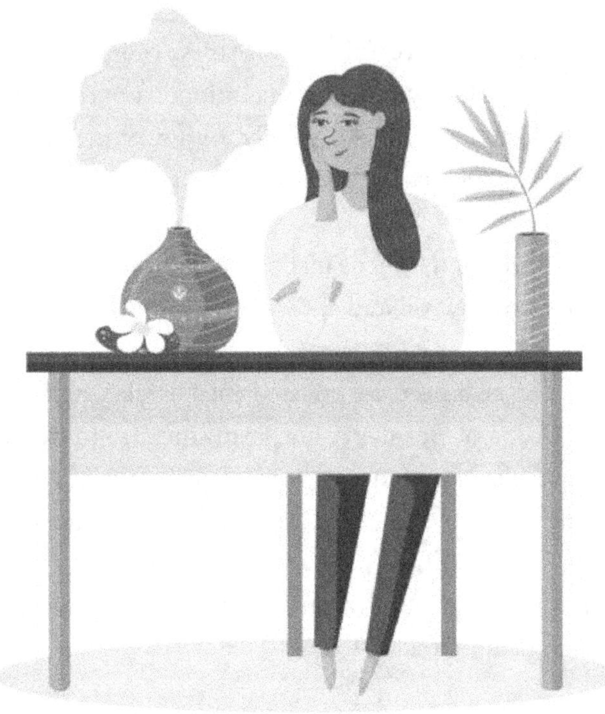

Essential oils can also be used to support immune health. Since Tea Tree and Eucalyptus, like mentioned earlier, are known for their antimicrobial properties they can be diffused in the home during cold and flu season. A simple immune-supporting blend for the diffuser could include a few drops each of Tea Tree and Eucalyptus oils together.

By incorporating essential oils into everyday routines, beginners can experience the profound benefits these natural wonders have to offer. Whether it's for personal care, household cleaning, stress relief, or overall health, essential oils can help enhance quality of life in a multitude of ways. The practical, hands-on approach of this chapter, combined with the specific examples and targeted information, aims to empower beginners to confidently and effectively use essential oils in their daily lives.

Nine

Essential Oil Recipes

Here are five simple blends to help you manage stress and anxiety

Serenity Blend

- 3 drops Lavender essential oil
- 2 drops Bergamot essential oil
- 1 drop Frankincense essential oil

I*nstructions:* Use in a diffuser or add to a carrier oil for a calming massage.

Tranquil Bath Soak

- 1 cup Epsom salts
- 1/3 cup Baking soda
- 2 drops Chamomile essential oil
- 3 drops Ylang Ylang essential oil

Instructions: Add to a warm bath for a soothing and relaxing experience.

Citrus Burst

- 3 drops Lemon essential oil
- 2 drops Orange essential oil
- 1 drop Peppermint essential oil

Instructions: Diffuse to create a refreshing atmosphere that uplifts and eases tension.

Grounding Blend

- 2 drops Vetiver essential oil
- 2 drops Cedarwood essential oil
- 1 drop Patchouli essential oil

Instructions: Use in a personal inhaler or diffuse for a sense of grounding.

Relaxation Roller Blend

- 10 ml Jojoba oil (or any carrier oil)
- 3 drops Lavender essential oil
- 2 drops Roman Chamomile essential oil

Instructions: Roll on wrists, temples, and pulse points for on-the-go stress relief.

Remember to personalize these recipes based on your preferences, and always perform a patch test before applying directly to the skin. Incorporate these blends into your daily routine for a natural and aromatic approach to stress and anxiety management.

Here are 3 essential oil blends that are often used for promoting health and well-being:

Immune Support Blend

- 2 drops of Tea Tree essential oil
- 2 drops of Eucalyptus essential oil
- 2 drops of Lemon essential oil

Instructions: Diffuse this blend during the cold and flu season to support a healthy immune system.

Digestive Harmony Blend

- 3 drops Ginger essential oil
- 3 drops Peppermint essential oil
- 2 drops Fennel essential oil
- 2 drops Orange essential oil

Instructions: Dilute this blend with a carrier oil and massage onto the abdomen in a clockwise motion for digestive support. The combination of Ginger, Peppermint, Fennel, and Orange can aid in promoting digestive harmony.

Respiratory Health Blend

- 2 drops of Peppermint essential oil
- 2 drops of Eucalyptus essential oil
- 2 drops of Rosemary essential oil

Instructions: Diffuse this blend to support respiratory health and ease breathing.

Remember: Always use high-quality, pure essential oils, and adjust the ratios based on personal preference. It's advisable to consult with a healthcare professional, especially if you have any existing health conditions or are pregnant.

Here are four essential oil blends for skincare that you can incorporate into your routine:

Nourishing Face Oil Blend

- 4 drops of Lavender essential oil
- 3 drops of Frankincense essential oil
- 3 drops of Rose essential oil
- 2 drops of Geranium essential oil
- Carrier oil (such as jojoba or sweet almond oil)

Instructions: Mix the essential oils with a carrier oil and apply a few drops to your face. This blend is known for its skin-nourishing and anti-aging properties.

Calming Skin Tonic

- 3 drops of Chamomile essential oil
- 3 drops of Lavender essential oil
- 2 drops of Patchouli essential oil
- 2 drops of Ylang Ylang essential oil
- Distilled water

Instructions: Mix the essential oils with distilled water in a spray bottle. Spritz on your face for a calming and soothing effect on the skin.

Acne-Fighting Serum

- 4 drops of Tea Tree essential oil
- 3 drops of Clary Sage essential oil
- 3 drops of Lemon essential oil
- 2 drops of Lavender essential oil
- Jojoba oil

Instructions: Mix the essential oils with jojoba oil and apply a small amount to areas prone to acne. This blend can help combat blemishes and promote clearer skin.

Hydrating Body Oil

- 5 drops of Neroli essential oil
- 4 drops of Rosemary essential oil
- 3 drops of Sandalwood essential oil
- 2 drops of Juniper Berry essential oil
- Carrier oil (such as sweet almond or coconut oil)

Instructions: Combine the essential oils with a carrier oil and massage onto damp skin after a shower for a hydrating and aromatic experience.

Always perform a patch test and dilute essential oils properly before applying to the skin. Adjust the ratios based on personal preference and skin sensitivity.

Here are five simple and effective essential oil recipes for cleaning:

All-Purpose Citrus Cleaner:

- 1 cup white vinegar
- 1 cup water
- 20 drops lemon essential oil
- 10 drops orange essential oil

Instructions: Mix all ingredients in a spray bottle. Shake well before use. Ideal for countertops, surfaces, and glass.

Tea Tree and Lavender Disinfectant Spray:

- 1 cup distilled water
- 1 cup rubbing alcohol
- 15 drops tea tree essential oil
- 10 drops lavender essential oil

Instructions: Combine all ingredients in a spray bottle. Shake well before use. Great for disinfecting surfaces and eliminating odors.

Eucalyptus Mint Bathroom Scrub:

- 1 cup baking soda
- 1/4 cup liquid Castile soap
- 10 drops eucalyptus essential oil
- 10 drops peppermint essential oil

Instructions: Mix baking soda and Castile soap in a bowl. Add essential oils and stir until a paste forms. Use for scrubbing bathroom surfaces.

Zesty Kitchen Degreaser:

- 1 cup distilled white vinegar
- 1 cup water
- 15 drops lemon essential oil
- 5 drops grapefruit essential oil

Instructions: Combine all ingredients in a spray bottle. Shake well before use. Perfect for cutting through grease on kitchen surfaces.

Lemon Fresh Floor Cleaner:

- 1 gallon hot water
- 1/2 cup white vinegar
- 20 drops lemon essential oil
- 10 drops tea tree essential oil

Instructions: Mix all ingredients in a bucket. Mop floors as usual. Leaves a refreshing and clean scent.

Remember to test these cleaners in inconspicuous areas before widespread use, especially on sensitive surfaces. Enjoy the fresh and natural scents while keeping your space clean!

Here are five energizing essential oil recipes that you can try:

Citrus Boost

- 3 drops of Lemon essential oil
- 2 drops of Orange essential oil
- 2 drops of Grapefruit essential oil

Minty Fresh

- 3 drops of Peppermint essential oil
- 2 drops of Eucalyptus essential oil
- 1 drop of Rosemary essential oil

Energetic Blend

- 2 drops of Bergamot essential oil
- 2 drops of Frankincense essential oil
- 2 drops of Ylang Ylang essential oil

Spice Up Your Day

- 3 drops of Cinnamon essential oil
- 1 drop of Clove essential oil
- 1 drop of Ginger essential oil

Forest Vibes

- 2 drops of Pine essential oil
- 2 drops of Cedarwood essential oil
- 1 drop of Juniper Berry essential oil

Instructions: Choose a recipe that resonates with you. Add the specified drops of each essential oil to your diffuser. Inhale the invigorating aroma and feel the energy boost.

Remember to adjust the ratios based on your personal preference, and enjoy the natural energy lift these blends provide!

Here are three kid-safe essential oil blends that you can use for children:

Good Morning, Good Day Blend

- 2 drops of Citrus Fresh essential oil
- 1 drop of Peppermint essential oil
- 1 drop of Sweet Orange essential oil

Instructions: Diffuse this blend in the morning to create a refreshing and invigorating atmosphere, promoting a positive start to the day.

Calming and Focus Blend

- 2 drops of Lavender essential oil
- 1 drop of Vetiver essential oil
- 1 drop of Frankincense essential oil

Instructions: Diffuse this blend during study sessions or times when focus and calmness are needed. It's a soothing and grounding combination.

Sweet Dreams Blend

- 2 drops of Chamomile essential oil
- 1 drop of Lavender essential oil
- 1 drop of Cedarwood essential oil

Instructions: Diffuse this blend in the evening to create a calming bedtime atmosphere, promoting a restful and peaceful sleep.

Always ensure that the essential oils used are kid-safe and suitable for children. Introduce new scents gradually and observe how your child responds. It's advisable to consult with a healthcare professional before using essential oils, especially if your child has any underlying health conditions.

Here are two pet-safe essential oil blends that you can use for a pleasant aroma without harming your furry friends:

Calming Blend

- 2 drops of Lavender essential oil
- 1 drop of Chamomile essential oil
- 1 drop of Frankincense essential oil

Instructions: Mix the essential oils and diffuse in a well-ventilated area. This calming blend can help create a relaxing atmosphere for your pets.

Fresh Citrus Blend

- 2 drops of Orange essential oil
- 1 drop of Lemon essential oil
- 1 drop of Spearmint essential oil

Instructions: Combine the essential oils and diffuse to add a refreshing citrus scent to your space. This blend can contribute to a lively and uplifting environment.

Always ensure that the essential oils used are pet-safe, and introduce new scents gradually to observe your pet's reaction. It's recommended to consult with a veterinarian before using essential oils around pets, especially if they have underlying health conditions.

Ten

Conclusion

In wrapping up our essential oil journey, let's recap the essentials we've covered. We started with the basics, learning about the history and science behind essential oils. Safety guidelines ensured our interactions with these oils were both enjoyable and secure. Exploring common and lesser-known oils gave us a diverse range of options to consider. Practical tips on buying and storing oils became our reliable guide. Finally, we honed in on seamlessly incorporating these oils into daily life, turning ordinary routines into fragrant moments. As we come to an end, take the knowledge gained and let it guide you towards a balanced lifestyle with the simple yet powerful influence of essential oils.

let's emphasize the core takeaways that will empower you on your ongoing essential oil journey. First and foremost, remember to adhere to safety guidelines when engaging with essential oils. This knowledge ensures not just enjoyment but also a secure experience with these potent extracts. Recognize that each oil has its own personality, offering specific benefits for various aspects of well-being. Lastly, integrate these aromatic wonders into your daily life deliberately. Whether it's enhancing personal care routines, transforming household cleaning, or simply finding moments of relaxation amidst the chaos, incorporating essential oils becomes a powerful tool for overall wellness and health benefits.

Now Let's reaffirm the myriad benefits that embracing essential oils can bring into your life. These aromatic extracts are not merely scents but powerful allies in shaping your daily experiences. Elevate your mood with the uplifting notes of citrus oils or find tranquility in the calming embrace of lavender. Harness the invigorating energy of peppermint to kickstart your day or create a sanctuary of relaxation with the soothing qualities of chamomile. Beyond their aromatic charm, essential oils contribute to improved health – from supporting skin vitality to aiding in respiratory well-being. Whether you're seeking a lift in spirits or support for your overall well-being, essential oils offer practical solutions for these everyday needs. If you need an energy boost, a mood lift, or a health perk, essential oils have your back.

It's essential to underscore the practical benefits that essential oils bring. Consider essential oils not as mere additives but as catalysts for holistic well-being. These aren't merely scents; they serve as tools for mood enhancement, increased energy, and improved health. Think of By weaving them into your routine, you're not just enjoying scents; you're tapping into their transformative power for improved well-being. Consider them integral elements in your routine, contributing to a balanced and harmonious life.

May this journey remind you of the practical advantages that lie within these tiny, aromatic bottles, ready to elevate your daily experiences.

<u>If you found this book helpful, please leave a favorable review on amazon so others can find it and benefit as well.</u>

Eleven

Resources

4 Ways To Tell The Difference Between Synthetic Oils And Essential Oils - Utama Spice. (n.d.). https://utamaspicebali.com/articles/4-ways-to-tell-the-difference-between-synthetic-oils-and-essential-oils/

Animals, M. F. (2023, July 25). *Which essential oils are toxic to pets?* Michelson Found Animals. https://www.foundanimals.org/essential-oils-toxic-pets/

Are essential oils safe for children? (2023, September 27). Johns Hopkins Medicine. https://www.hopkinsmedicine.org/health/wellness-and-prevention/are-essential-oils-safe-for children

Aromatherapy: Do essential oils really work? (2021, August 8). Johns Hopkins Medicine. https://www.hopkinsmedicine.org/health/wellness-and-prevention/aromatherapy-do-essential-oils-really-work

Butnariu, M., & Sărac, I. (2018). Essential Oils from Plants. *Journal of*

Biotechnology and Biomedical Science, 1(4), 35–43. https://doi.org/10.14 302/issn.2576-6694.jbbs-18-2489

Cronkleton, E. (2019, March 8). *Aromatherapy Uses and benefits.* Healthline. https://www.healthline.com/health/what-is-aromathe rapy#how-does-it-work?

Gomez, L. G. (2023, January 13). *Can you put essential oils in a humidifier?* Nikura. https://nikura.com/blogs/living-well/can-you-put-essential-oils-in-a-humidifier#:~:text=Add%20a%20few%20drops%20of,to%20v aporise%20around%20the%20room.

History of Aromatherapy:: International Federation of Aromatherapists. (n.d.). https://ifaroma.org/ko_KR/home/explore_aromatherapy/what -is-aromatherapy/history-aromatherapy

Keeping with Tradition: Essential Oil History, Use and Production: A Review. (2019, June 27). *Cosmetics & Toiletries.* https://www.cosmetics andtoiletries.com/cosmetic-ingredients/natural-sustainable/article/21 835552/keeping-with-tradition-essential-oil-history-use-and-product ion-a-review

Kelly, L. (2022, May 27). Essential oil storage tips: 5 Best practices to Increase oil Longevity. *Millstone Farm & Organics Inc.* https://millston eorganics.com/blogs/news/essential-oil-storage-tips-5-best-practices

Maker, M. (2022, February 26). *Everything you Need to Know About Cleaning with Essential Oils! - Clean My Space.* Clean My Space. https://c leanmyspace.com/cleaning-with-essential-oils/

mindbodygreen. (2018, May 18). *How To Make Essential Oils.* Mindbodygreen. https://www.mindbodygreen.com/articles/how-essential-oils-are-made

More, D., MD. (2022, March 10). *Can you be allergic to essential oils?* Verywell Health. https://www.verywellhealth.com/allergy-to-essential-oils-83218

OM Blend Aromatic Spritzer. (n.d.). JUSU - All Natural. Plant Based. Good for You and Good for the Earth. https://getjusu.com/products/om-blend-aromatic-spritzer

The distillation of essential oils. (n.d.). Pranarôm FR. https://www.pranarom.fr/en/content/15-the-distillation-of-essential-oils

The Editors of Encyclopaedia Britannica. (1998, July 20). *Essential oil | Uses, Types & Extraction.* Encyclopedia Britannica. https://www.britannica.com/topic/essential-oil

Woods, J. (2023, November 3). *13+ Essential Oils for Face Steaming | Steaming Guide, Benefits And DIY Recipes.* https://gyalabs.com/blogs/essential-oils/essential-oils-for-face-steaming

www.ingramcontent.com/pod-product-compliance
Lightning Source LLC
Chambersburg PA
CBHW060840260726

48661CB00002B/529